The Gym Rules

Your Guide To Navigating
The Gym Floor

By
Daniel Williams

Front cover image by Nookie Design
Illustrations by Nookie Design

Getoutfitness.co.uk

Disclaimer
The advice and strategies found within may not be suitable for every situation. This work is sold with the understanding that neither the author nor the publisher are held responsible for the results accrued from the advice in this book.

Special thanks

I would like to thank everyone who took it upon themselves to take time away from their gym session to comment, mention or complain to me about the state of the gym, other members or just needed to rant. All of you inspired me to bring all your thoughts into one book.

Introduction

For a lot of people, the gym is where we spend most of our free time. The gym has become part of the daily routine, many people wake up early before sunrise to go to the gym and get in a workout before heading to work. Others head straight from work to the gym often not getting home until very late, just in time to eat the evening meal and go to bed. There are few who manage to get a workout done during their lunch breaks, it's not really much of break though!

We can't escape fitness; it is all over the media. Every time we turn on the TV, someone is selling us a gym membership or selling us a product to help get fit quick. Celebrities promote their very own fitness DVDs 'Get Your Beach Body in just Six Weeks' or something along those lines. Social media apps like Instagram and Twitter are full to the brim with fitness enthusiasts who can get 100,000 likes from posting a gym selfie. We spend so much time engrossed in and around fitness, it has taken over our lives.

This book aims to help you get a better experience while trying to keep fit and healthy.

With all this time we spend working out, it's inevitable that we will come across something or someone that irritates us, or maybe you are the person that irritates others. If you are the latter then this book is defiantly for you.

This book comes from a career of working in gyms as well as being a gym member myself. Issues that have come up while working with clients, observations of other members and conversations with fellow instructors. This book also comes out of frustration, frustration of what often goes on in some gyms. The following pages are broken down into rules or guidelines that will help everyone co inhabit the places that a lot of us call the second home.

50 rules/guidelines, detailing how to get a better experience from the gym or avoid the culprits that may ruin your precious time.

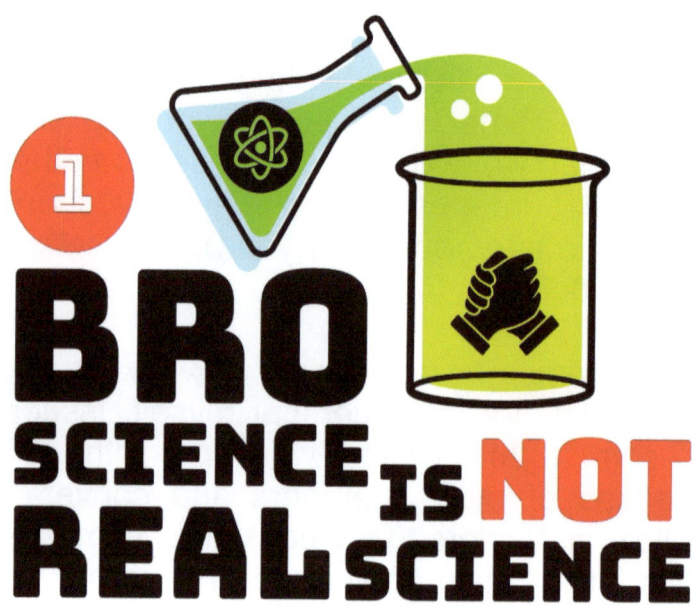

BRO SCIENCE IS NOT REAL SCIENCE

1

Bro Science is often an opinion rather than fact-based evidence with regards to fitness and nutrition. The general belief of "it worked for me Bro, it will work for you too!" or "my mate told me, who heard of a friend who knows this crazy strong bodybuilder...... so it must be true" is why opinions are accepted over facts. Not all Bro Science is false, but Bro Science advice should be taken with caution. It is very easy these days to find research papers on all subjects, especially nutrition. That said, interpreting data correctly is tricky and this is why it should be left to the people who have actual PHDs.

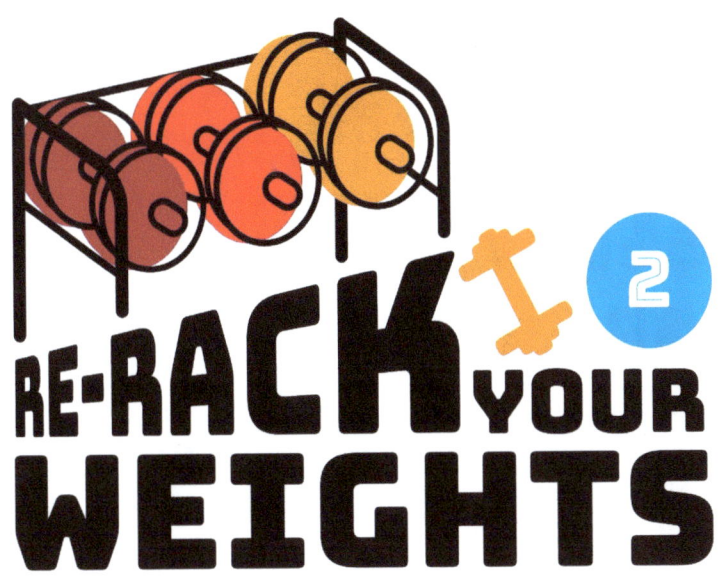

RE-RACK YOUR WEIGHTS

It is not the responsibility of the gym staff to clean up after you. If you really want to hit those fitness goals then get that little extra pump by picking up the weights and re-rack them. Respect the gym, Respect the gym equipment.

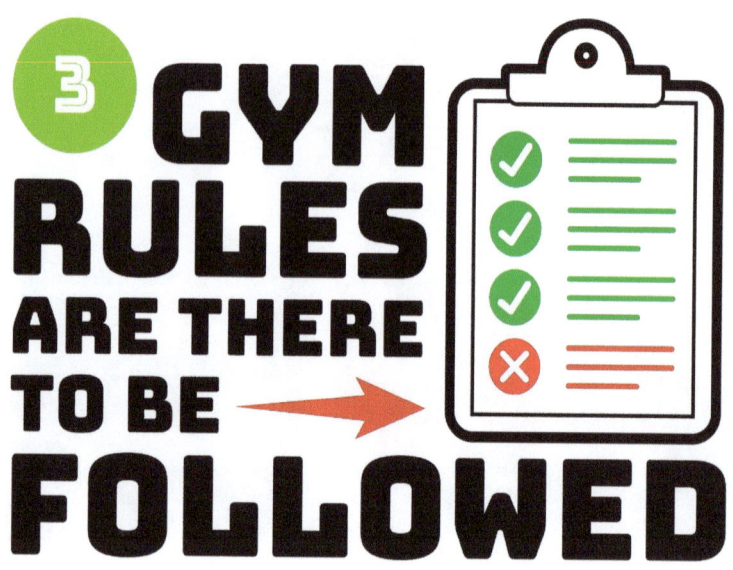

3 GYM RULES ARE THERE TO BE → FOLLOWED

The same way your office or work site has rules, so does the gym. They are not recommendations. A lot of them are for health and safety reasons. Remember gym equipment is often heavy and can cause serious harm and even death.

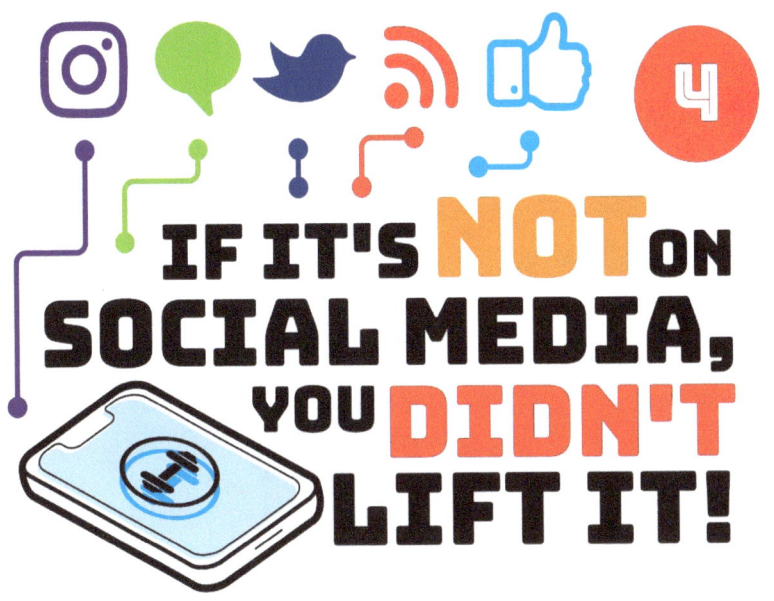

IF IT'S NOT ON SOCIAL MEDIA, YOU DIDN'T LIFT IT!

We have all heard the story about how your friends' mates uncles cousin managed to squat 1 million lbs for 50 reps or how a friend who knows a guy who once lifted a 100kg dumbbell over his head without warming up. Well over 5billion people have phones, one of those people could have recorded the epic gym achievement and posted it on some social media site for the world to see!

If not, it didn't happen.

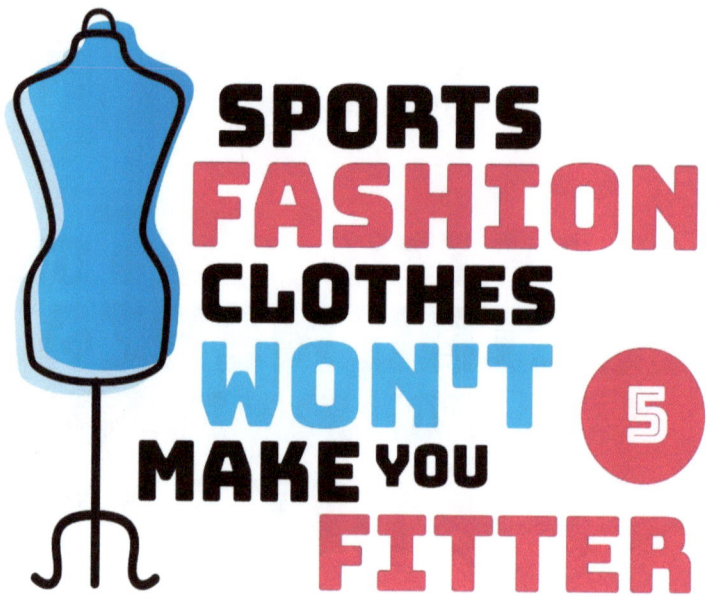

SPORTS FASHION CLOTHES WON'T MAKE YOU FITTER

5

There is nothing wrong with wanting to look good, for sure that is one of the main reasons we workout, right? But if you spend more time and effort on what you wear to the gym then when you go on a night out, you need to question your intentions. Is it to get fitter or to impress?

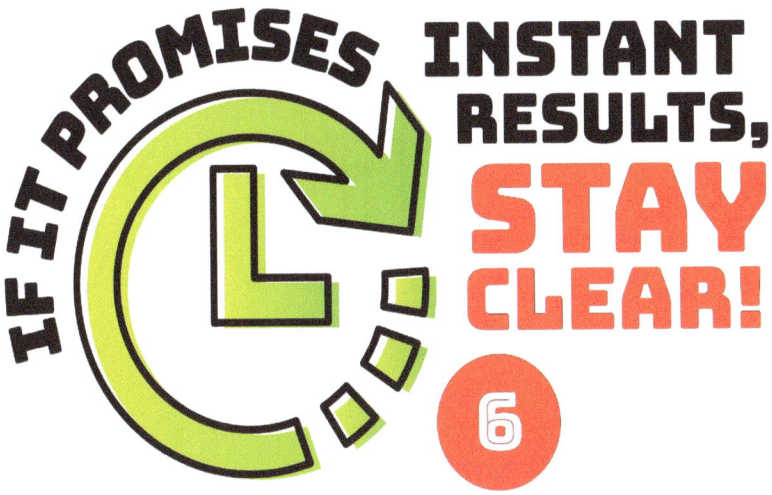

IF IT PROMISES INSTANT RESULTS, STAY CLEAR!

6

There is no quick fix in fitness, no magic pill that will transform your body. If there was then there would be no need for gyms and the world would be a sexier place. Fitness takes effort, dedication and often the drive to push through the pain barrier. You can't gain muscle or lose fat overnight, it takes months sometimes years to reach those goals.

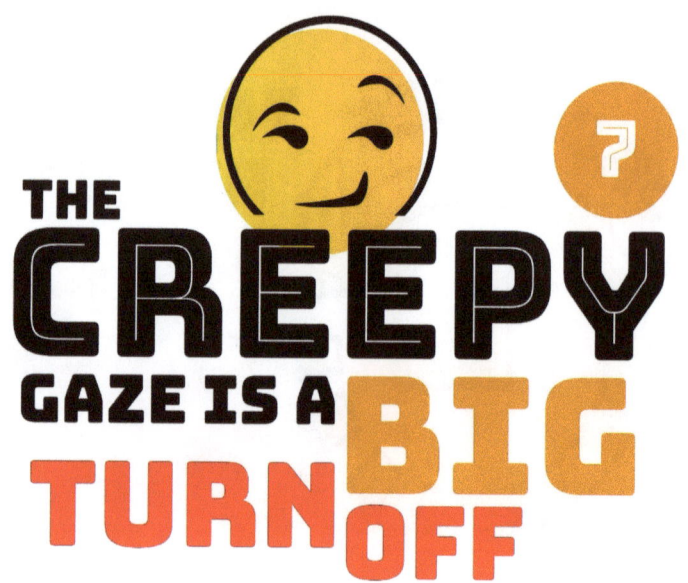

THE CREEPY GAZE IS A BIG TURN OFF

This rule is directed mainly at the men. Prolonged staring at the opposite sex is creepy and off putting to the recipient. There is nothing wrong with noticing someone who is attractive, it's human nature. But to openly stare at someone at length is un-called for and is seen as repulsive and obnoxious by others. Gyms can be very intimidating for some people and the last thing they need is someone making them feel even more uncomfortable.

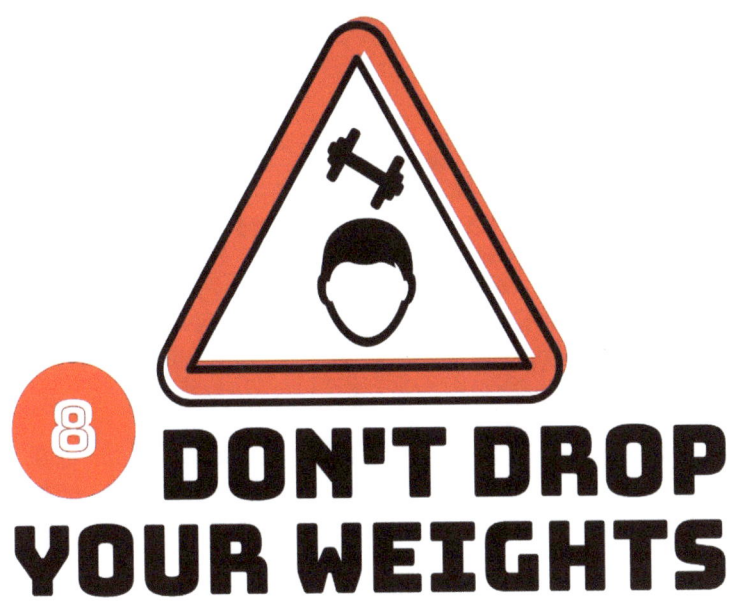

DON'T DROP
YOUR WEIGHTS

Dropping weights is not a sign of strength, it's a sign of disrespect. There are a few exceptions, if there is a risk of injury, you are a power lifter in the Olympics or you attend a CrossFit box. Some strongman events, dropping weights will result in a 'no lift/failed attempt'. So, if the strongest man in the world can manage to put down the weights without causing a raucous, then surly everyone else can.

9 DON'T TALK TO SOMEONE WHILE THEY ARE TRYING TO DO THEIR REPS

Interrupting someone mid-set is not only disrespectful, it is also dangerous. A lapse of concentration can result in severe injury, so if you need to say something to someone, either wait until the end of their set or get their attention by getting into their line of sight. Side note, head phones are seen as a sign as 'do not disturb'!

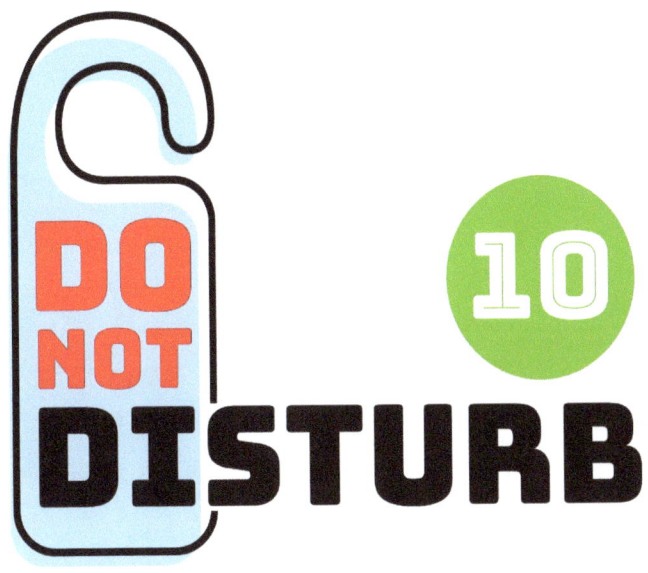

This rule follows on from rule 9. If someone is wearing headphones or earphones then take it as a sign that they wish not to be disturbed. A friendly nod of the head or wave is fine, but unless they reach for the headphones, to remove them, say no more and carry on with your workout.

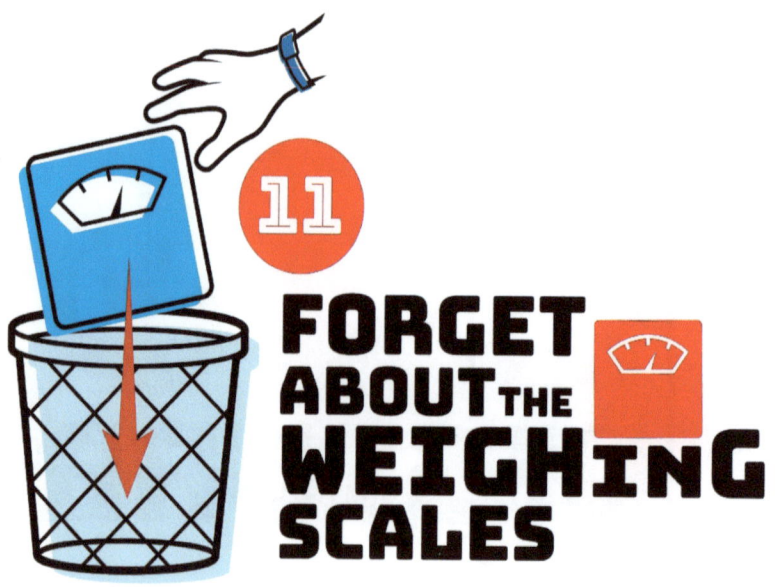

FORGET ABOUT THE WEIGHING SCALES

There are three main factors to consider when working out:

1) How you feel.
2) How you look.
3) Your weight.

If you been working out a while and you feel good within yourself, feel stronger and fitter, look better in the mirror and your clothes are fitting better or feeling loose why do the scales mean so much? There is no magic number to weigh in at. Why not forget the scales and concentrate on how you look and feel instead?

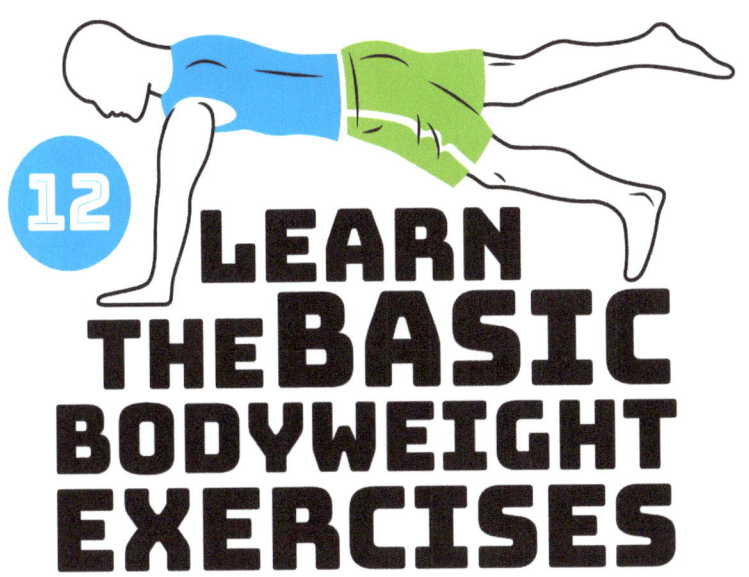

12 LEARN THE BASIC BODYWEIGHT EXERCISES

Learning the key bodyweight movements; push ups, pull ups, dips, squats and sit ups will enable many things. Firstly, it allows you to work out almost anywhere, anytime, in a park, at home or maybe a hotel room to name a few. Learning to work with just bodyweight will help reduce stress loads on joints. Another good factor to bodyweight exercises is that there are so many variations to all the basic movements you can always keep the workouts creative.

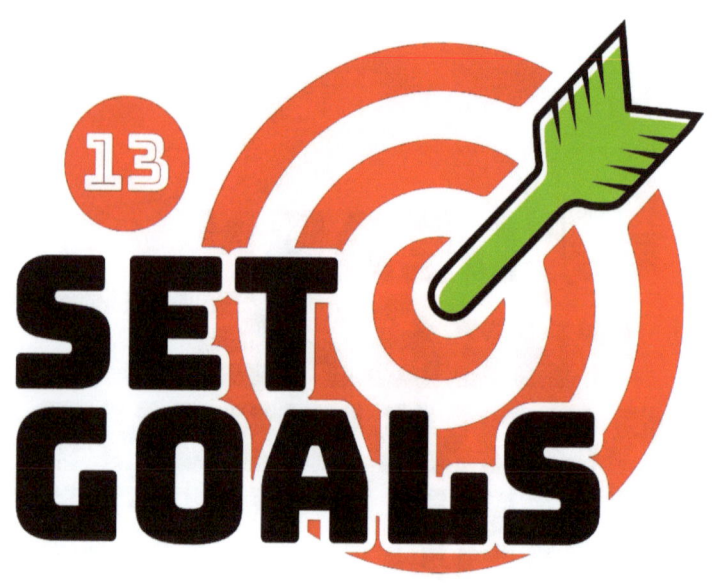

13 SET GOALS

Goal setting is a great way to stay motivated. Make sure the goals are realistic though. Popular goals are getting beach ready for holidays, to be able to fit into a certain outfit or drop a dress size. With goal setting try and set smaller, easily achievable goals that will lead to your main goal.

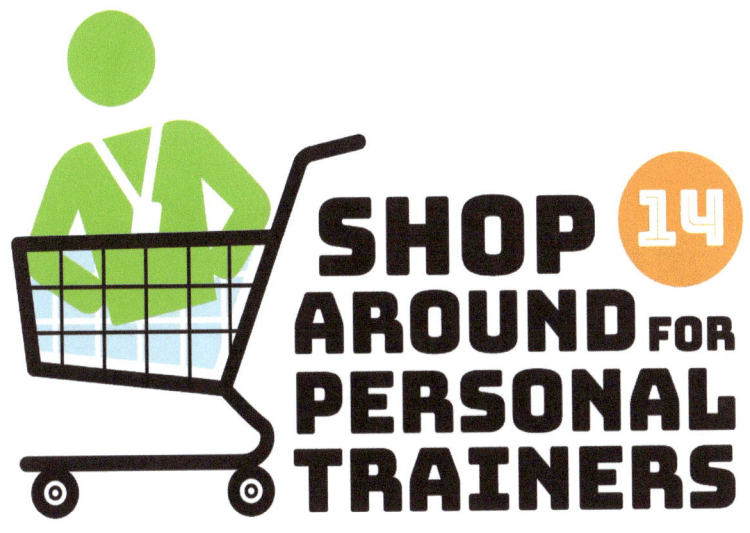

SHOP 14 AROUND FOR PERSONAL TRAINERS

Not all personal trainers are the same. Like in all other professions there are good trainers and bad trainers. Some will be money grabbing and will only tell you what you want to hear, others will give you the truth even if it's not what you want to hear. Some have great interpersonal skills, others may struggle to engage with you. You need to be confident in your personal trainer and be able to get on with them. Don't just go with the first one you see or fancy.

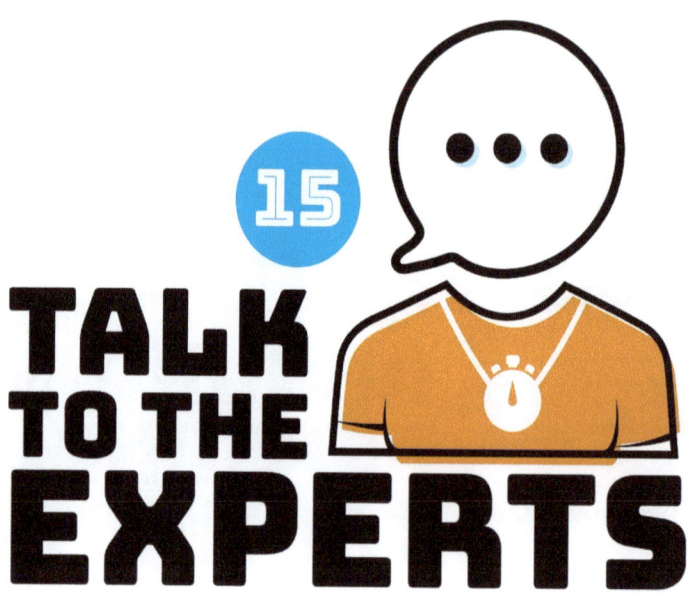

TALK TO THE EXPERTS

15

Sure you can try and fix your car yourself, but it will take a hell of a long time and you will most likely get a few things wrong before you get it right. Instead you simply take your car to the mechanic and leave it in the hands of the professionals. Treat your body as a car. Seek expert advice, they can guide you in the right direction a lot quicker and more efficiently.

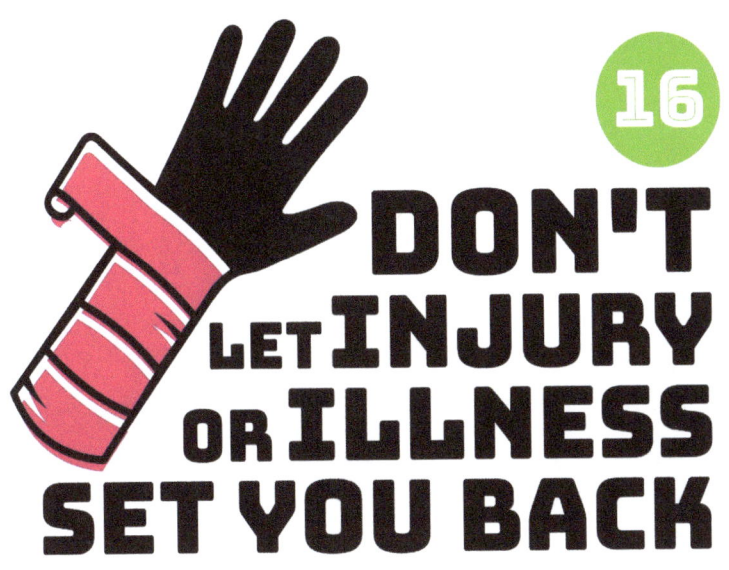

DON'T LET INJURY OR ILLNESS SET YOU BACK

16

At some point everyone gets an illness or an injury, but don't let it setback training any-more than it needs to. Rest, recover, refocus, and return. The longer time spent away from fitness the harder it gets to return, physically and mentally.

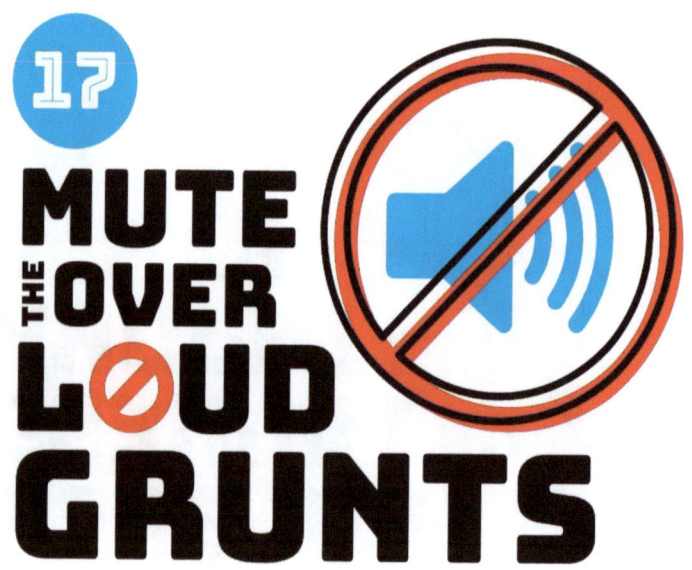

17

MUTE THE OVER LOUD GRUNTS

It is understandable you want to psych yourself up. But do you need to let the whole gym know that you are going to lift some weights. The same goes for people who grunt on every single rep, tone it down.

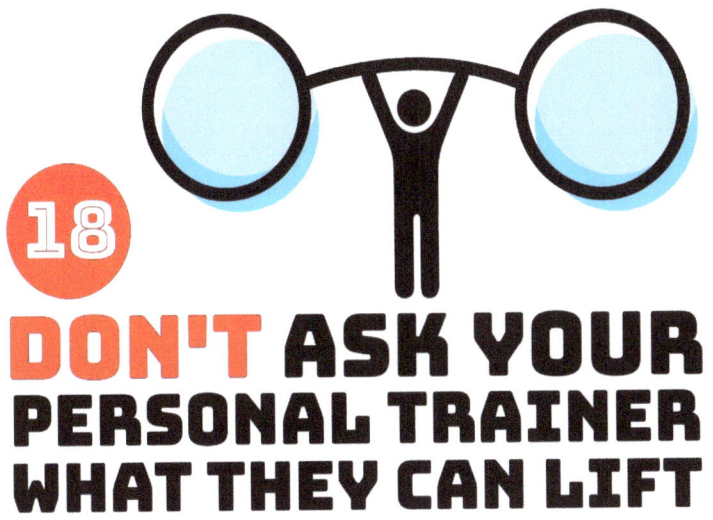

18
DON'T ASK YOUR PERSONAL TRAINER WHAT THEY CAN LIFT

Personal trainers basically live in the gym, so they have an advantage when it comes to working out. So, it should come as no surprise that most will be fitter then the average person. A personal trainer is there to help people reach their health and fitness goals, and a personal trainer should be able to perform the exercises they prescribe, but it can be demoralizing to the client if the fitness levels are hugely apart SO DON'T ASK!

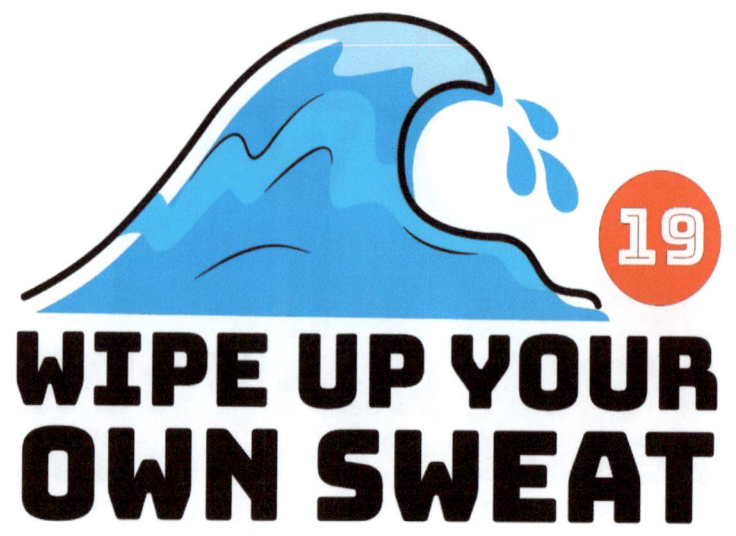

WIPE UP YOUR OWN SWEAT

There is only one time that most people want to be in contact with other people's sweat and when we do, we tend to know the other person very personally. Sweat is made up of water and trace amounts of chemicals including ammonia. Yes, sweat is basically urine. So, in the purpose of hygiene make sure you take a towel or wipe down gym equipment with paper towels after use.

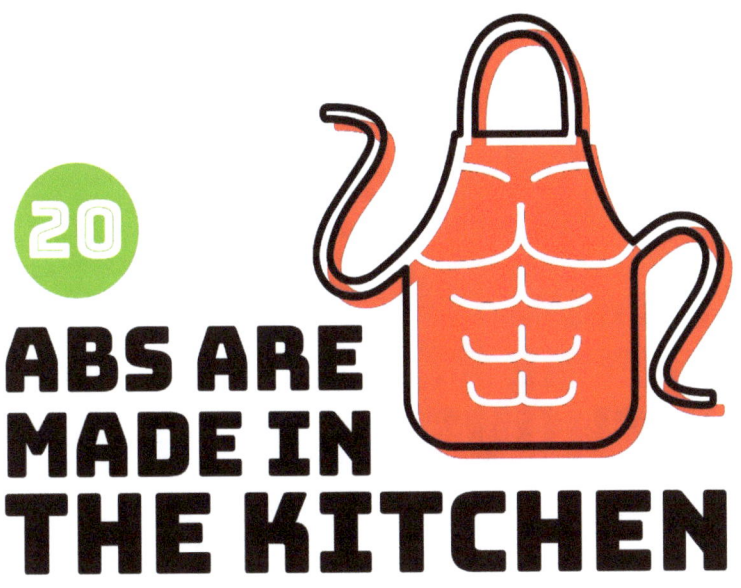

20

ABS ARE MADE IN THE KITCHEN

It doesn't matter how many sit ups you knockout each day; you won't see your abs underneath a thick layer of fat. The only way to see them is to get that body fat percentage down. Most men need to achieve a body fat percentage of six to nine percent; women need to reach 16 to 19 percent body fat. A healthy, balanced nutrition plan is the key to reaching those low levels of fat. Not just exercise.

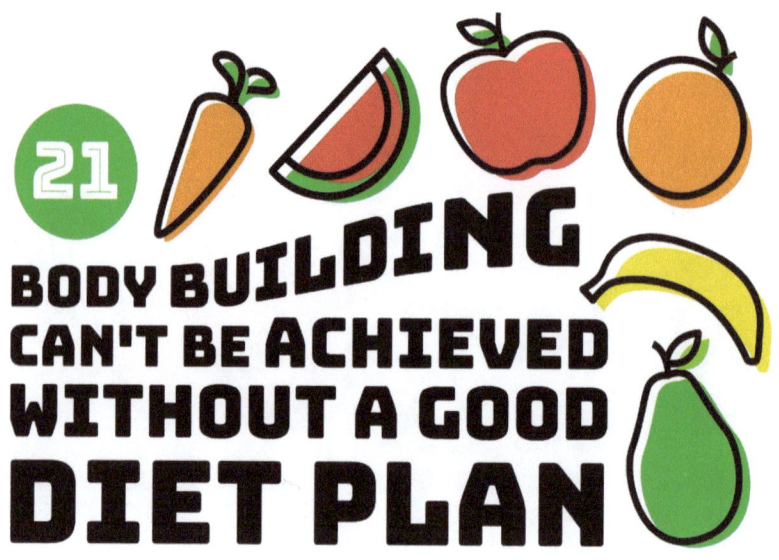

21 BODY BUILDING CAN'T BE ACHIEVED WITHOUT A GOOD DIET PLAN

Everyone knows that to lose weight you need to create a calorie deficit, so the body burns more calories than it consumes. The key to bodybuilding is not simply to lifts lots of weights but to also fuel the body correctly. A balanced blend of complex carbohydrates, complete proteins, and fats, combined with how you eat and when you eat will greatly affect how the muscles will grow. Not eating enough will result in little to no progress. Eating lots of junk food will result in huge levels of body fat, covering the muscles.

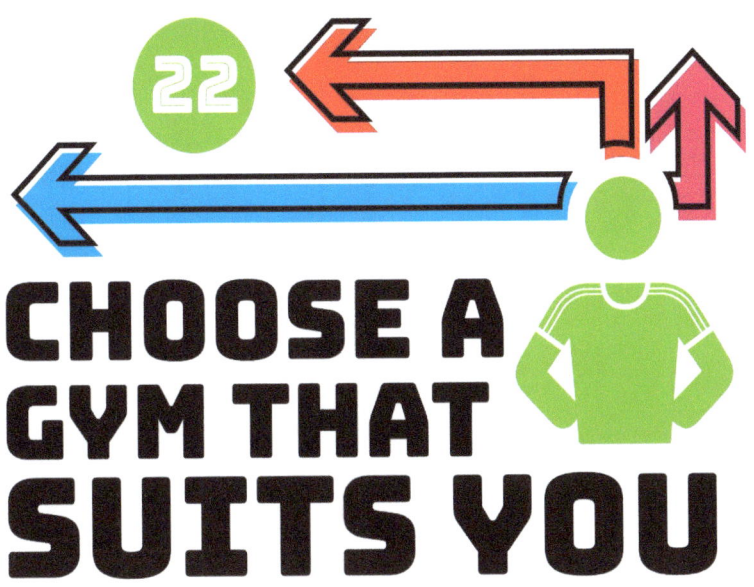

CHOOSE A GYM THAT SUITS YOU

There are so many types of gyms these days, budget gyms, leisure centre, spas, strongman gyms, outdoor bootcamp companies. Find out what you enjoy doing and find a gym that caters for your needs. The closest or cheapest may not always be the most suitable.

IF YOU HAVE A GYM MEMBERSHIP, USE IT!

Its takes much more than just having a gym membership to get fit. Regular attendance is a good starting point. So many people never step foot in the gym after the first month of their membership but will carry on paying the monthly fees, sometimes for an entire year or longer. Gyms are very happy to take the public's money, even more so if you don't even use the facilities. Basically, you are giving money away for nothing if you don't use your membership.

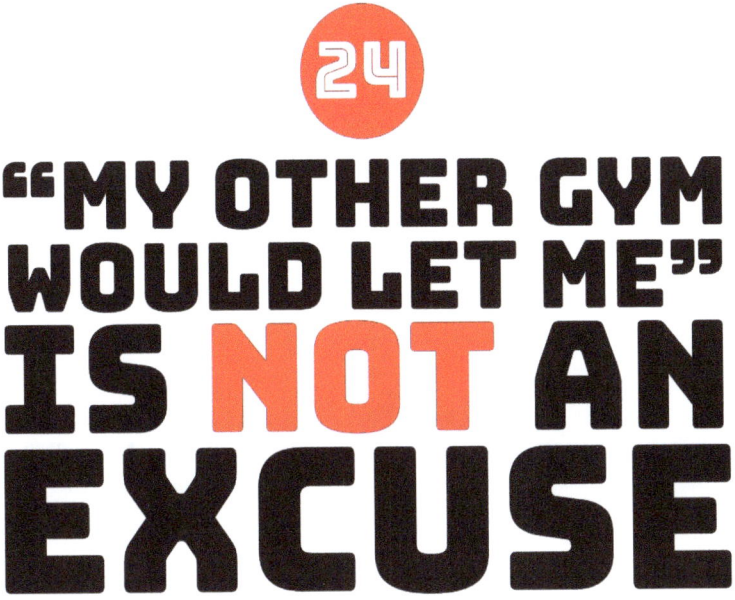

24

"MY OTHER GYM WOULD LET ME" IS NOT AN EXCUSE

This means nothing the current gym staff. If your other gym was so much better then maybe you should cancel your current membership and return to the good old glory days where you can do whatever you like.

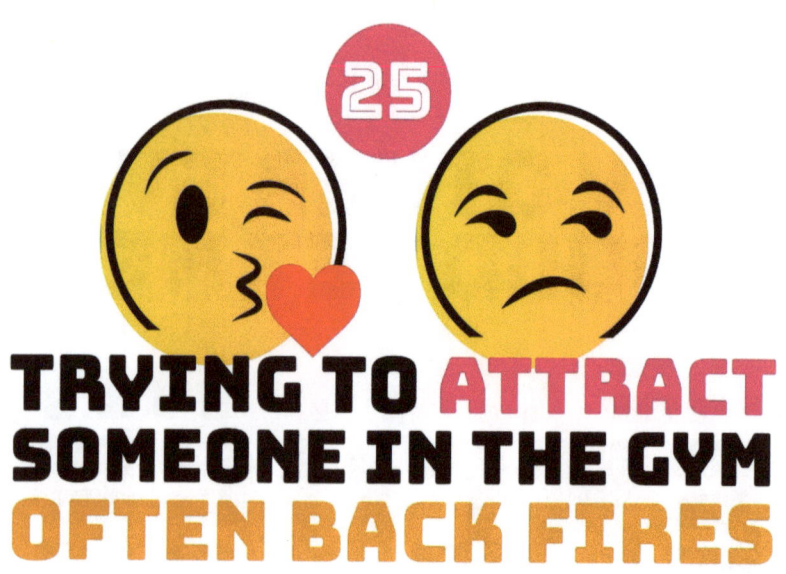

TRYING TO ATTRACT SOMEONE IN THE GYM OFTEN BACK FIRES

They say that one of the best places to meet a potential partner is in the gym. You already have something in common, keeping fit and staying healthy, but be careful. Gyms are small communities where a lot of people talk. Don't be the one that everyone is talking about, the one that sleeps or tries to sleep with everyone and anyone. You could quickly find yourself ostracised and looking for a new gym to join.

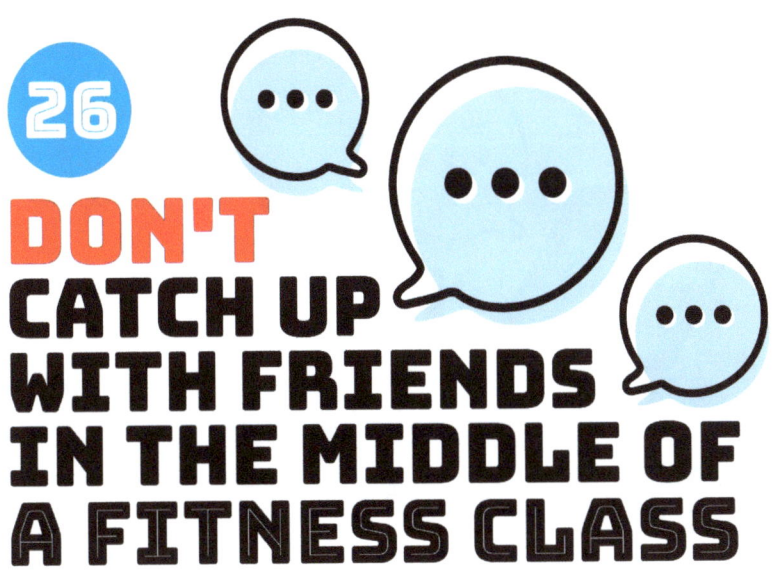

26
DON'T CATCH UP WITH FRIENDS IN THE MIDDLE OF A FITNESS CLASS

Friends love to do classes together, it's a great motivational tool to get to the gym. But don't chat over the instructor while they are telling the rest of class what exercises you are going to be doing. It is rude and makes you look like a naughty school kid at the back of the class. Why not wait till the end of the class so you can a proper catch up.

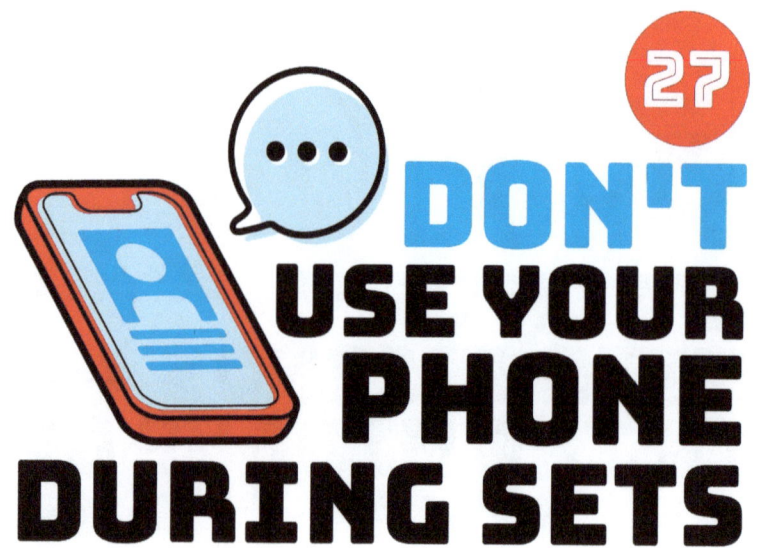

DON'T USE YOUR PHONE DURING SETS

Can you not live without your phone for roughly an hour? If you can't then try only using your mobile in-between sets. There is no way you can lift weights effectively and talk on your mobile. If you are not concentrating on the exercise, you are not pushing the muscles hard enough, which will result in no physical change in the body.

I'M USING THAT, MATE!

If you see a towel or drinks bottle on a piece of equipment then it's normally a clear sign that it's in use. Be polite and do a quick ask if anyone is using a particular piece of equipment.

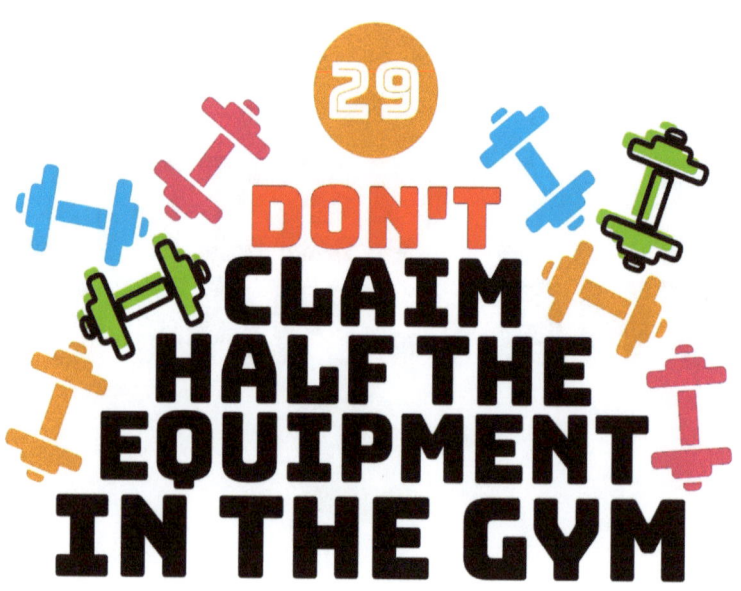

29
DON'T CLAIM HALF THE EQUIPMENT IN THE GYM

Sometimes we like to perform circuit-based workouts that require multiple pieces of equipment. If that is the case then try and do these kinds of workouts in off peak times when the gym floor is a little quieter. Don't start claiming the dumbbells, squat rack, bench press, TRX and every other piece of equipment in the middle of peak times. Other people need to work out as well.

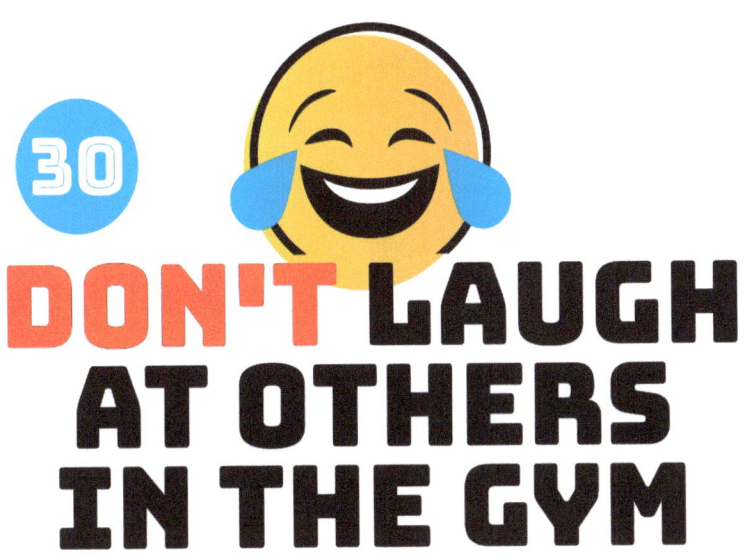

DON'T LAUGH AT OTHERS IN THE GYM

We are not all fitness gods in the gym. Remember people go to the gym to get fitter and healthier, don't give someone a hard time because they may be overweight or not using the equipment correctly. That fat guy you laughed at could turn out to be one of your fitness peers. If someone is using a piece of equipment incorrectly, then inform a member of staff or if you have the knowledge, go and politely correct them.

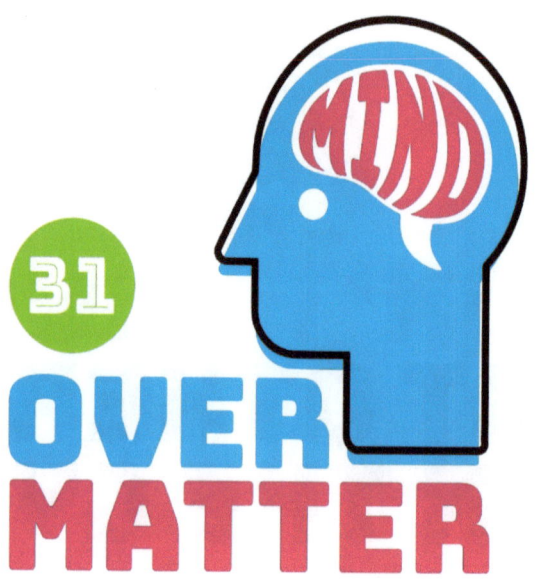

31 OVER MATTER

The body can achieve so much if encouraged by the mind. One of the main factors in achieving a goal is not the physical challenge but the mental challenge. People often put a limit on what they can achieve and the body will work up to that limit, or until the mind says otherwise. Instead of setting a challenge of what you think you can do, set a challenge to see what you can do! Here is an example for people lifting weights. Ask your training partner to load the weights for you, without telling you what the weight is. Often people will lift a higher amount of weight than they thought possible.

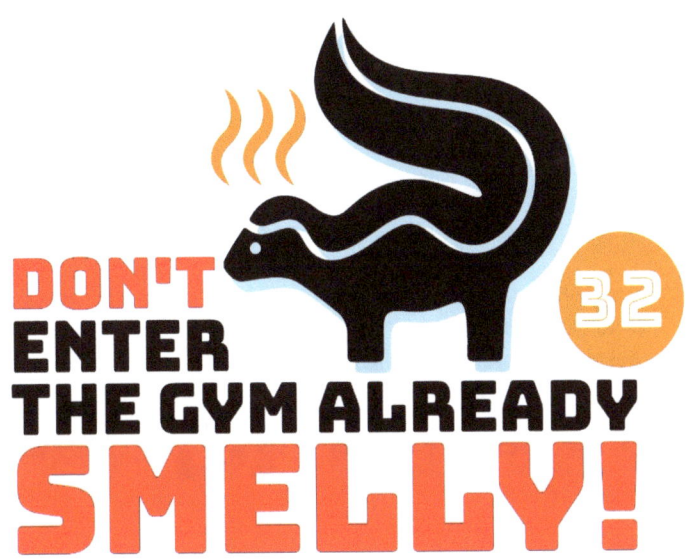

DON'T ENTER THE GYM ALREADY SMELLY!

32

There is nothing wrong with leaving the gym smelling of sweat, but there is no excuse to enter the gym already stinking. You may have a stressful or demanding job but use the showers before getting changed into gym attire.

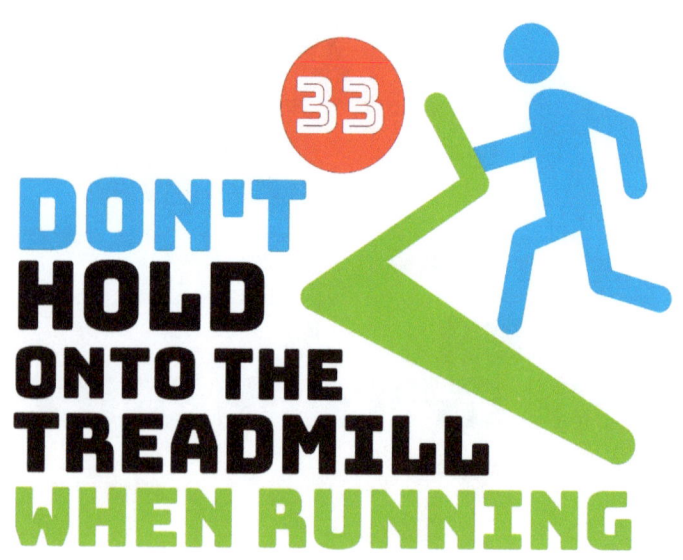

DON'T HOLD ONTO THE TREADMILL WHEN RUNNING

33

We don't hold onto handrails when walking or running outdoors, so unless you have coordination or balance issues, there is no reason to hold the hand rails on a treadmill. Firstly, holding onto the rails drastically reduces the workload placed on the body resulting in an easier workout and fewer calories burned. Secondly, holding onto the rails creates a muscular imbalance, the body isn't allowed to move freely which can lead to tension in the hips, shoulders and back resulting in potential muscular strain injuries.

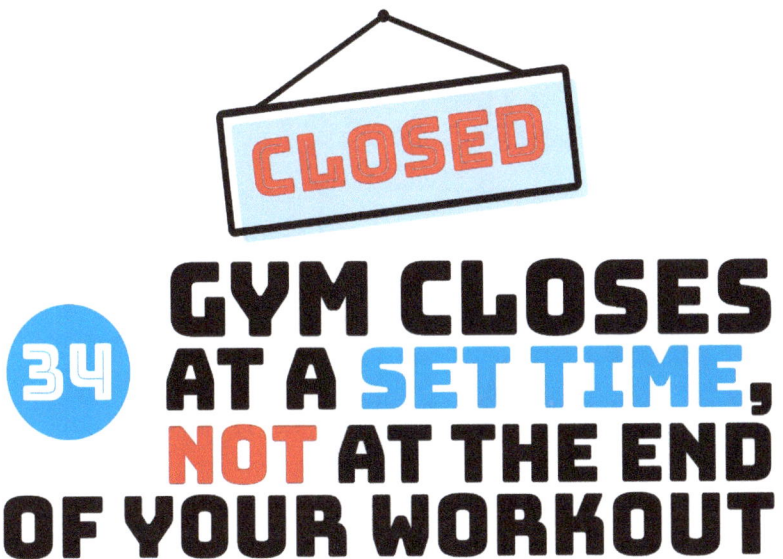

GYM CLOSES AT A SET TIME, NOT AT THE END OF YOUR WORKOUT

34

Everyone likes to workout at different times of the day but don't arrive at the gym 30 minutes before it closes expecting to do a 1 hour workout. No matter how much you argue about the need of your gainz, the gym will still close at the same time as the night before.

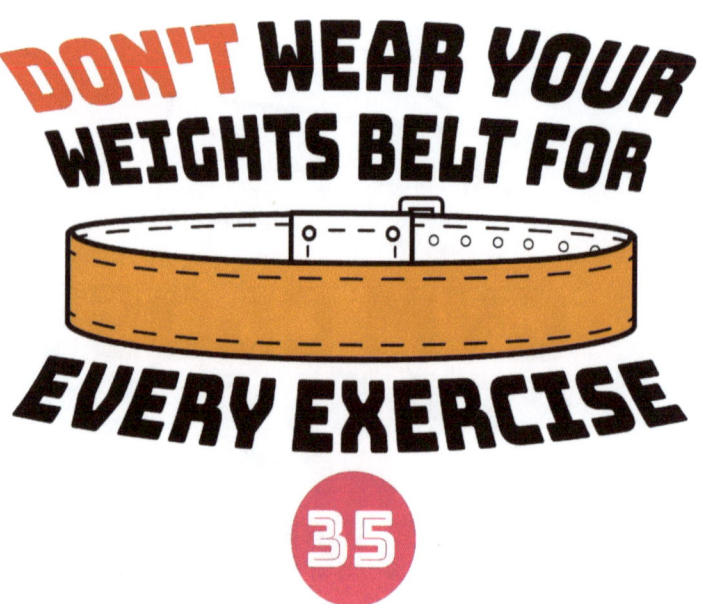

DON'T WEAR YOUR WEIGHTS BELT FOR EVERY EXERCISE

35

The weights belt is a great tool for lifting heavy loads that place pressure on the lower back. That is it! It's not a fashion accessory! If you need to wear a weights belt to do light lifts or exercises like 'cable triceps push downs' then you have a core problem and maybe you should do more core-based exercises to strengthen that area.

EMBRACE DE-LOAD WEEKS

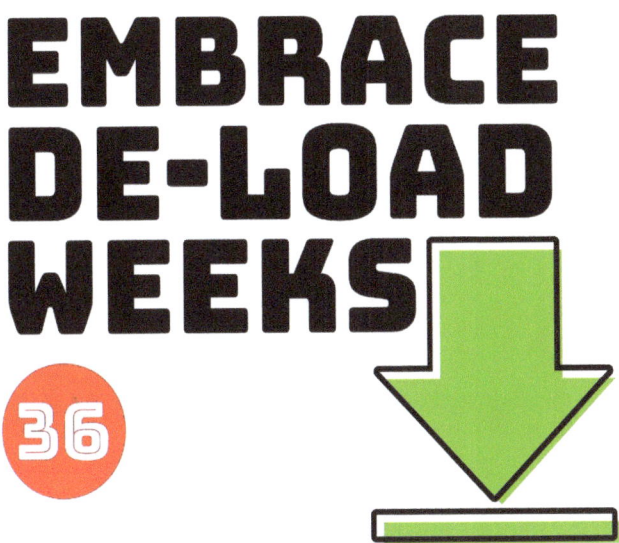

36

You should take a deload week between weeks 6-8 or 12-14 of your workout programme. They are essential for everyone who works-out on a regular basis, from high performance athletes to everyday gym-goer. Deloading allows the mind and body to recover and refocus, helps overcome plateaus and reduces the chance of injury.

There are 3 ways to deload:

1) Lower the intensity of the exercise, ideally around half of what you would normally lift.
2) Lower the volume of the exercise, only a couple of repetition per set.
3) Change the workout completely, if you lift a lot of weights then go for runs or bike rides and vice versa.

Take a break, it will do you good.

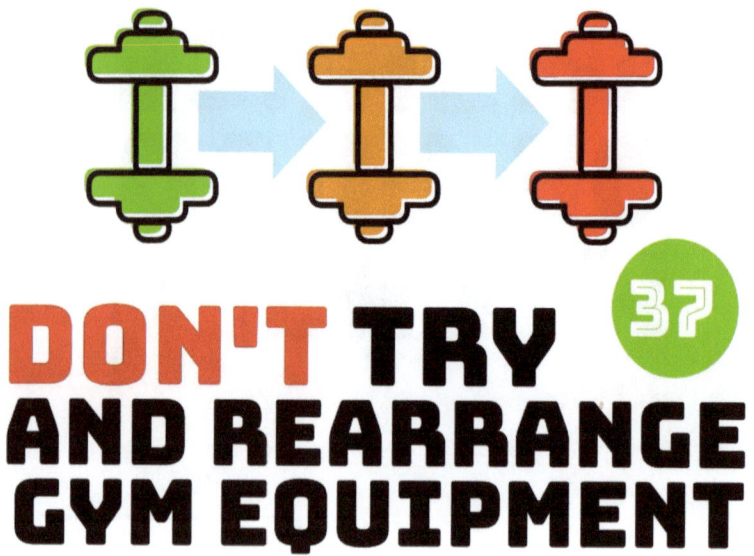

DON'T TRY AND REARRANGE GYM EQUIPMENT

Each gym has its own layout. For better or for worse, leave the heavy equipment where it is. Just because you can move the weights around it doesn't give you permission to move the bench press.

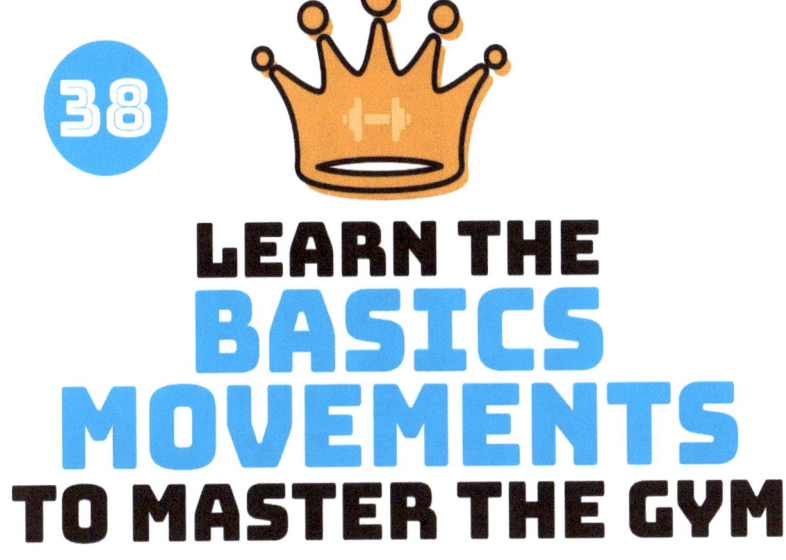

38

LEARN THE
BASICS
MOVEMENTS
TO MASTER THE GYM

There are 5 basic exercises that everyone should know and do in the gym, deadlift, squat, bench press, dips and pull ups. There are so many variations of these 5 movements that you can continuously keep changing your workout programme indefinitely. Learn them!

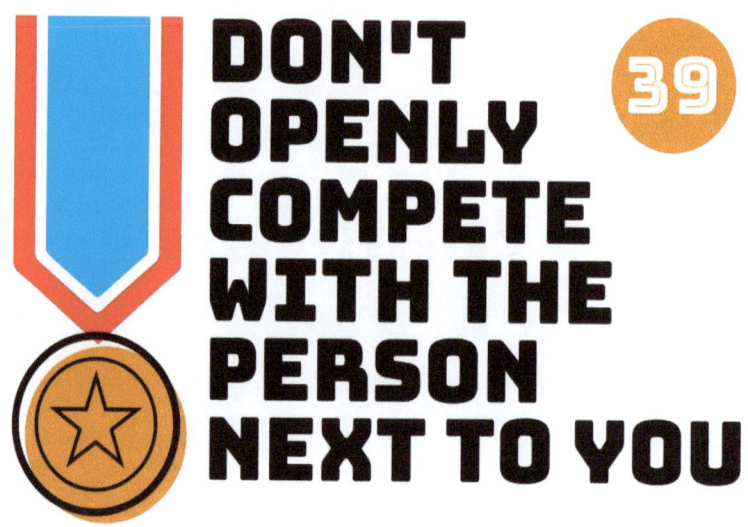

DON'T OPENLY COMPETE WITH THE PERSON NEXT TO YOU

39

We all like a challenge and nothing motivates us more than being pushed by someone else. But there is no need to jump on the adjacent treadmill and compete with someone who is just doing their own workout. Wait until they have finished, ask them what kind distances they run, for how long? They will openly share with you their training goals, most people do. Then afterwards, try and beat it, Or better still get a training partner that you can have a friendly competition with.

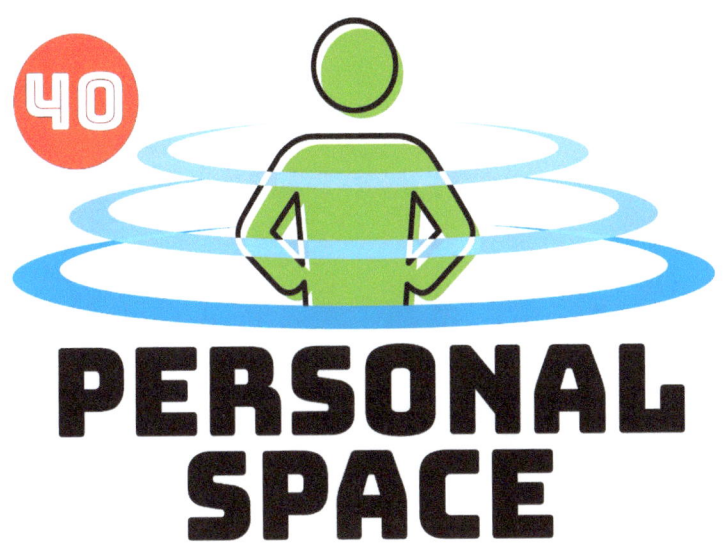

PERSONAL SPACE

Unless the gym is bursting at the seams with members, you don't need to stand directly next to another member. Remember, to exercise you need to move, which often results in arms swinging out to the sides or in front or the legs going out in many directions. You don't want to get accidentally hit, or worse be thought of as a gym creep so step back a little bit.

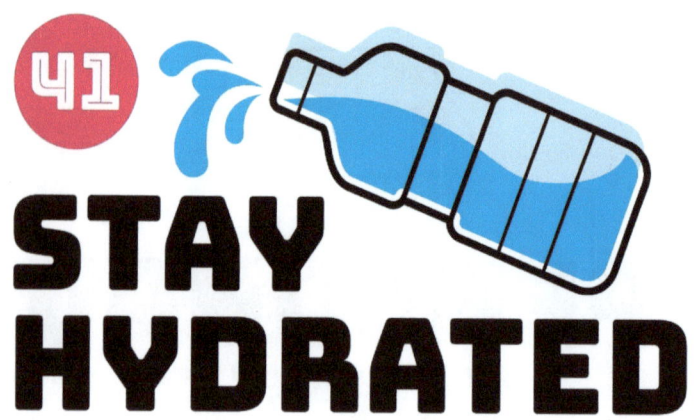

STAY HYDRATED

The benefits of drinking water and staying well hydrated are amazing. It keeps the brain working at peak effectiveness, it helps flush toxins out the body. Staying hydrated can help with weight loss. A lot of people can't tell the difference between being hungry and thirsty and often mistake thirst for hunger, which results in over eating. Staying hydrated throughout the day will help keep hunger at bay.

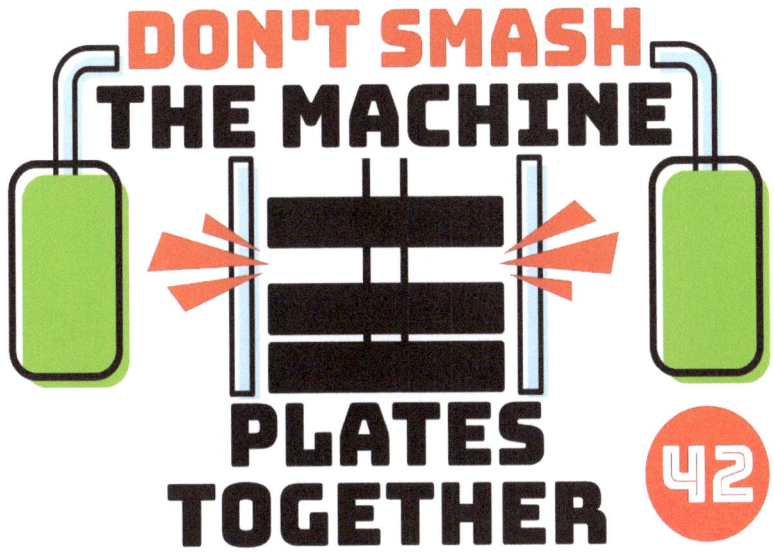

DON'T SMASH THE MACHINE PLATES TOGETHER

42

The weights may be cast iron but the components are not. Often, they are held together with small screws. They break easily but are difficult to reach and replace. No one cares that you can lift heavy and no one wants to hear about it when you do. You don't have to finish you set with a literal bang. Respect the equipment.

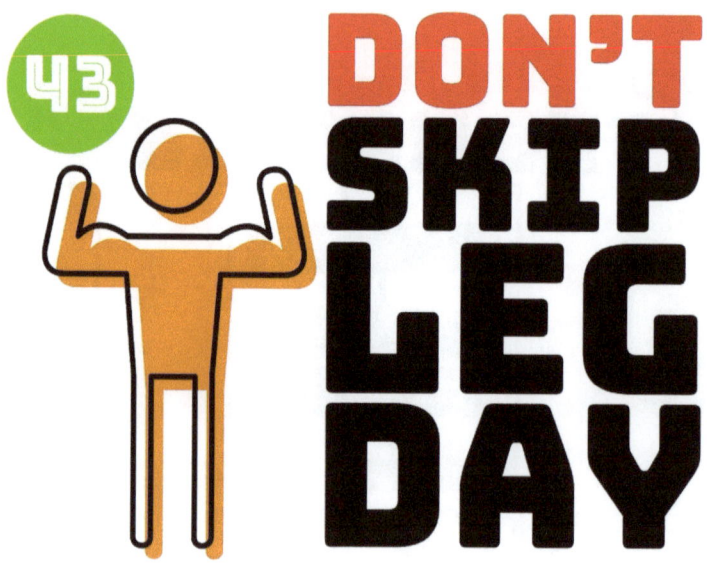

This goes for any muscle group, skipping workouts because they are hard is ill advised. The benefits will outweigh the short term pain. Missing sessions on the same set of muscles will also create a muscle imbalance, which never looks good aesthetically and can lead to injures.

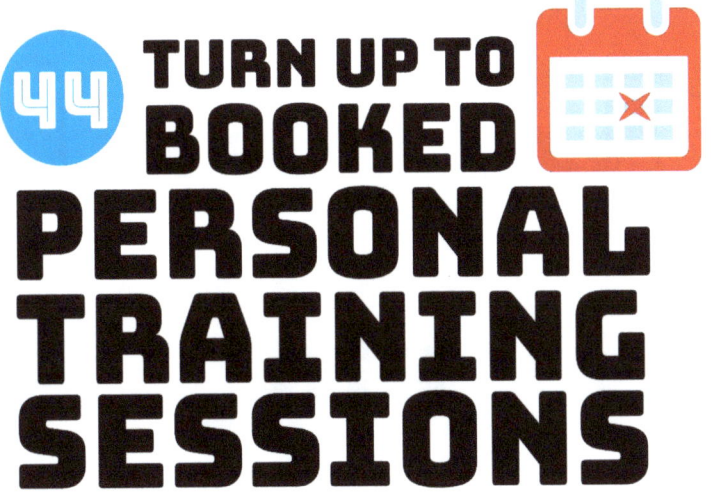

44 TURN UP TO BOOKED PERSONAL TRAINING SESSIONS

Sometimes people need to rearrange bookings and meetings, this also happens for personal training sessions. With a bit of notice (normally 24hrs), a personal trainer will happily rearrange a PT session, as long as it's not a weekly occurrence. It is not okay to cancel 5 minutes before or worse not show up at all without an excuse. Because this happens far more than it should most gyms and personal trainers have written agreement with clients, where the client is still charged for the session if cancelled within 24hrs of appointment.

You wouldn't skip out on a work meeting, don't do it for personal training sessions.

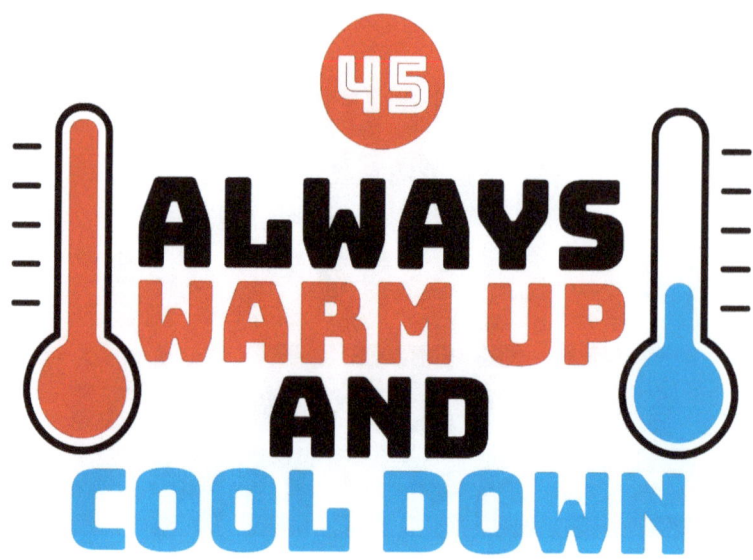

45
ALWAYS WARM UP AND COOL DOWN

Warming up and cooling down are as essential to the workout as the workout itself. The warm up helps minimise the risk of injury and prepares the joints to work under load through the full range of motion. To do this you want to oxygenate the muscles and insure the ligaments and tendons are well lubricated with synovial fluid. To achieve this, a light cardio-based movement is advised followed by some dynamic stretches for 5-10 minutes.

Cool downs are to allow the body to return back to normal. Not cooling down, especially after a vigorous workout can result in blood pooling in the legs, which can lead to light headiness, dizziness, nausea and fatigue. Light jogging to a slow walk, keeping the arms below the heart is ideal.

Static stretching will help relive any tension built up in the muscles, 30 second holds are advised for all the major muscle groups.

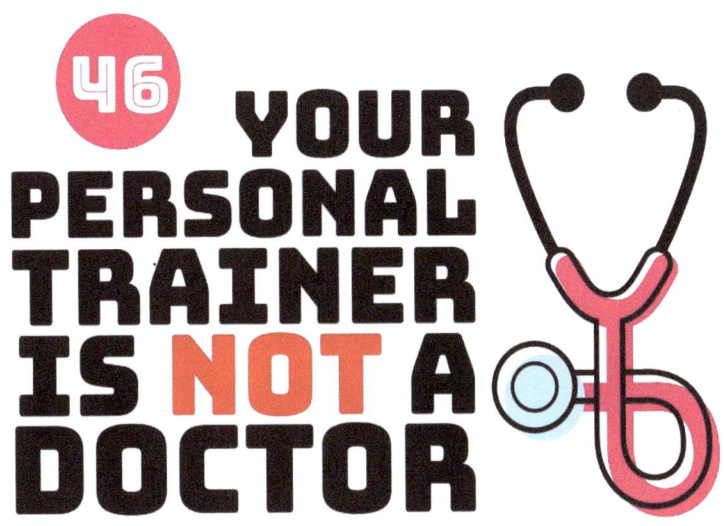

46 YOUR PERSONAL TRAINER IS NOT A DOCTOR

A good personal trainer understands how the body works physically. He or she is trained to help the public become fitter and healthier through the means of exercise, nutritional advice and lifestyle choices. A personal trainer is not doctor and is not qualified to diagnose any symptoms presented to them. If you experience any physical ailments, visit your doctor or physiotherapist first.

USE IT OR LOSE IT

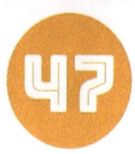

There is no clear cut answer to the question "How quickly will I lose it"? A lot can depend on why you have taken a break from fitness in the first place, if it was due to injury or not, what level of fitness you had in the first place, plus the type of fitness you do. Fitness deteriorates at different rates with regards to strength and cardio. According to various studies a loss in 20% of V02 max can be seen in a just 4 weeks. Studies have also shown that muscle fibres can show no change upwards of 4 weeks however sports specific strength can start to decline in as little as two weeks.

On the plus side, if you were fit in the first place, it is much easier to regain your fitness again.

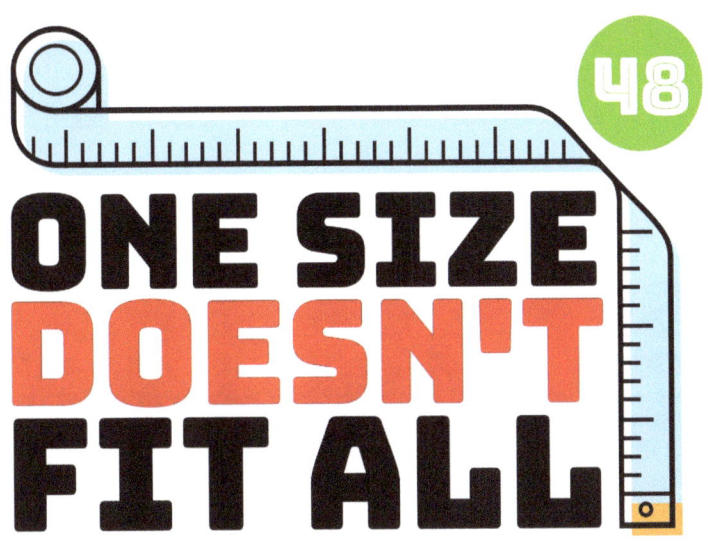

ONE SIZE DOESN'T FIT ALL

We all know that one guy in the gym who just has to look at the weights and he suddenly packs on 3 kilos of pure muscle! You copy what he does but for some crazy reason you don't see the same gains.

There are so many different ways to workout, circuit training, super sets, German volume training to name just a few. Often a lot of them will produce the same results. The defining feature to all workouts is you, the individual. We all respond differently, sometimes in huge ways, sometimes just smaller changes.

Find what works for you.

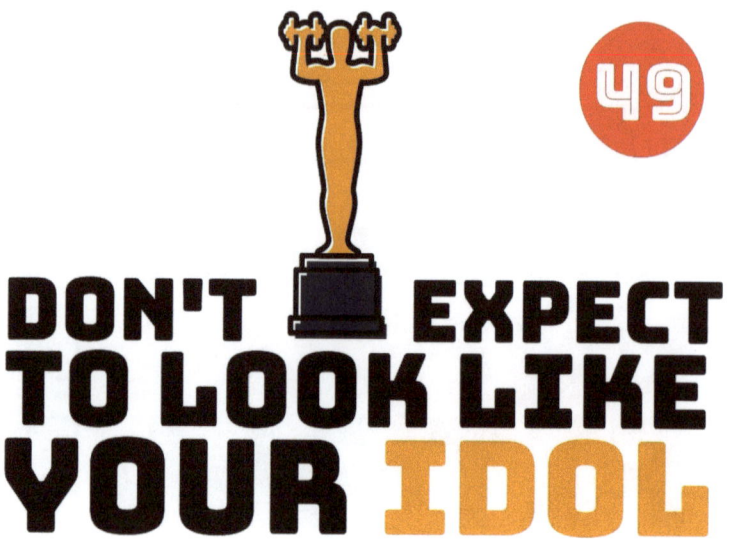

DON'T EXPECT TO LOOK LIKE YOUR IDOL

This rule leads on from, the "One Size doesn't fit all rule". If you idolise The Rock (Dwayne Johnson) and follow his training programme and nutritional plan to the letter, but you start looking like Danny DeVito don't be surprised if you don't look the mirror image of The Rock. Your height and body frame play an important role in your overall look.

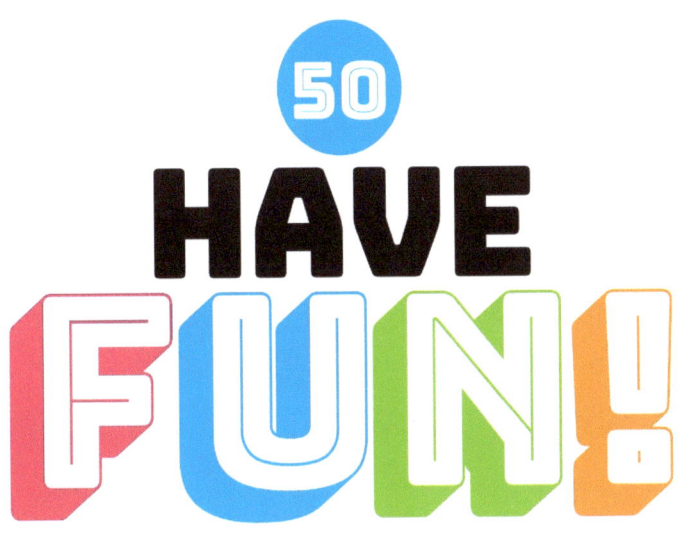

50

HAVE FUN!

This rule is often over looked when it comes to working out. Nobody is forcing you to the gym so why are you there if you don't enjoy it? There are so many different ways to keep fit, take up a sport, join a club, workout with friends or workout outdoors. Do what you enjoy!

www.ingramcontent.com/pod-product-compliance
Lightning Source LLC
Chambersburg PA
CBHW040746010626
45792CB00027B/301